MY PREGNANCY DEVOTIONAL JOURNAL

My Pregnancy Devotional Journal

40 Weeks of Reflection and Prayer for You and Your Baby

KYTIA L'AMOUR

Illustration by Jacinta Kay

ROCKRIDGE PRESS

Interior and Cover Designer: Stephanie Sumulong
Art Producer: Sara Feinstein
Editor: Carolyn Abate
Production Editor: Andrew Yackira
Production Manager: Riley Hoffman
Author photo courtesy of Jerrell Conner

Illustration © 2021 Jacinta Kay
Author photo courtesy of Jerrell Conner

Paperback ISBN: 978-1-63807-376-5
R0

To my husband, Jerrell; my angel baby in heaven; and my two children, Petra and Olivier. I wouldn't be who I am today if God hadn't blessed me with all of you.

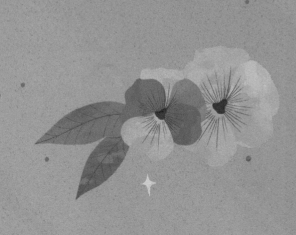

Contents

Introduction

Welcome to your pregnancy devotional journal! However you got here, I'm glad to have you and to be able to walk you through 40 weeks of your motherhood journey. Whether this is your first time becoming pregnant or you already have a growing tribe, this is a special time and there's no other experience like it! Moms have drastically different journeys with each baby, and your faith itself matures and grows with every new child. What's unique about this devotional is that you get to see how your daily life *and* walk with God are impacted by this special person (or people!) soon to enter the world.

I'm blessed to have two incredible children who proved to be much different from each other in the womb and outside of it. Through each new symptom and circumstance, what helped me the most in both pregnancies was prioritizing my time with Jesus. It's no wonder women tend to cling to the Word of God the most during this stage of life—I mean, pregnancy is kind of a big deal! Motherhood impacted my faith in such a phenomenal way, and I hope the lessons I share in this book will help you just as much in your relationship with Christ and pregnancy in general.

As a mother, you might tend to internalize your questions, memories, and prayers. With this book as your guide, you can get those thoughts down on paper—and remember them for years to come. Isn't it wonderful that the baby in your womb may actually get to read this one day? Each devotional begins with an encouraging and edifying scripture to meditate on throughout the week, followed by a lesson diving deeper into the meaning of the passage and suggestions on ways to apply it to your life. Then, you have a chance to coauthor with me. By answering journal prompts, recording a memory, and saying a prayer over your life, you can customize this book as much or as little as you desire.

There's no fruit chart included in this journal to track your baby's growth, but the topics will organically coincide with what you might be dealing with in each stage of pregnancy—physically, emotionally, and spiritually. This includes the "fourth trimester," when your baby is a newborn. Most women don't discover they're pregnant until they are about six weeks along, but the 40 devotionals included here will still be pertinent to your week-to-week experience. Also, if a topic doesn't hit home right away, then skip it and come back to it later when it feels more applicable.

As you make your way through the lessons, keep these helpful practices in mind:

→ Take your time. You have an entire week for each entry.
→ Read alongside your Bible for more scriptural context.
→ Be as brief or as thorough in your entries as you'd like.

Let's get started—I can hardly wait!

A New Creation

> *Your eyes saw my unformed body;*
> *all the days ordained for me were written in*
> *Your book before one of them came to be.*
>
> **PSALM 139:16 (NIV)**

I remember a few days after finding out I was pregnant with my son, my five-year-old daughter asked me a version of "Where do babies come from?" I figured this topic would come up at some point in her life, but it didn't fail to make me blush. I paused and answered, "Daddy and I prayed and asked God to bless us with a new baby, and He decided now was the right time."

Of course, there is more to how babies are conceived, but the role that prayer plays is important. Whether your pregnancy was a surprise, a difficult journey, or a somewhat planned event, the truth remains the same: Only God creates life and decides when it will begin. I imagine Him having a conversation with each of us before He sends our spirit into a human body. I think of how He might tell us who our family is and what our calling will be as He prepares us for our lifetime on Earth.

You might be feeling mixed emotions about your pregnancy. Even if you've had kids before, I can tell you with certainty that this child will provide a unique experience. Something that brings me peace as a mother is knowing that God has a plan, and nothing is a surprise to Him. From the moment of conception to the time when we reunite with Him in heaven, He knows every choice we will make, every mistake, every triumph, and every hurt.

At times when you feel ill-equipped to parent this precious gift, know that God chose you specifically to carry this child and take on the responsibility of raising them with His help. This is a moment to trust, surrender, and rest in God's strength.

How does it feel knowing that God chose you specifically to care for this child? Understanding God is co-parenting with you, how do you now see your responsibility as a mother?

_____

_____

_____

_____

_____

_____

_____

What are some of your hopes and dreams for this child's life?

_____

_____

_____

_____

_____

_____

_____

_____

What was your initial reaction to finding out you were pregnant? Be detailed about those emotions so you can look back clearly on that experience years from now.

_____

_____

_____

_____

_____

_____

_____

_____

God, please help me surrender my anxiety to You as I embark on this joyous and blessed journey. (Continue your prayer here.)

_____

_____

_____

_____

_____

_____

_____

Your Reward from Heaven

> *Children are a heritage from the Lord,*
> *offspring a reward from Him.*
>
> **PSALM 127:3 (NIV)**

Roughly 44 percent of all pregnancies around the world are unplanned. In fact, if you've announced your pregnancy to anyone, then one of the first questions to come up is "Was this planned?"

Sadly, there's often a negative connotation to unplanned pregnancies. But you and I know that God calls each child a blessing no matter how they got here. For those of you who were surprised by a positive pregnancy test, you may feel it's taboo to express your excitement after the shock wears off. I say it's natural to be excited about and feel love for your unborn child, whether this is your first or an unexpected sixth baby.

When friends of ours told their family that baby number four was on the way, the mood quickly went from excitement to worry. Concerned relatives asked if this would be the last one, hinting the couple should stop having so many children.

Unfortunately, some people can be quick to put their preferences on others. Perhaps family members, friends, or even coworkers don't want a large family because it would be too much, so they raise their own concerns to families who seem to be adding a new child each year.

Other people may praise couples who stop at one boy and one girl, calling it "the perfect combination." Whatever your preference or circumstance, continue to be thankful for the blessing that is new life, and ask God to help you raise them well.

Have you ever had other people place their preference on you regarding family planning? How did you deal with that?

_____

_____

_____

_____

_____

_____

_____

How has this pregnancy already impacted your life in a positive way?

_____

_____

_____

_____

_____

_____

_____

_____

What were the initial reactions when you announced
your pregnancy?

_____

_____

_____

_____

_____

_____

_____

Father, please continue to help me see this child as a blessing in
my life and to raise them well. (Continue your prayer here.)

_____

_____

_____

_____

_____

_____

_____

_____

Birthing the Next Generation

> *Like arrows in the hands of a warrior are children born in one's youth. Blessed is the man whose quiver is full of them.*
>
> **PSALM 127:4-5A (NIV)**

There are so many wonderful scriptures detailing children as blessings, rewards, and gifts. Children are also a great asset in the battles we face in life. The Psalm passage here describes children as arrows, and what a blessing it is to have a quiver full of them. I'm not by any means telling you that God wants you to have 12 children, but there is a reason we're told in the book of Genesis to be fruitful and multiply.

The purpose of having children isn't simply to line up our offspring and show them off in order to prove how much God loves us. It's not to ensure we have someone to take care of us when we get older. The purpose of children is to raise them in God's strength and truth; the generation we raise will become some of the greatest Christ followers we have the privilege of serving alongside.

I see the simile of children as arrows, shot against the enemy, as a bolt of purpose, moving at lightning speed to dismantle humanity's worst tendencies. I see bondage broken, generational curses removed, and God's hand freely moving in your bloodline.

It can be difficult to parent when you think about the state of the world and worry about the challenges your children might face. But I remind myself, like Esther, that they were born for such a time as this. Raise your children in the teachings of Christ, and they will become the answer to many of the world's troubles and a beacon of hope for those in despair.

How can you be intentional about helping raise a strong generation of Christ followers?

_____

_____

_____

_____

_____

_____

_____

_____

What are some of the ways you can incorporate the knowledge of Jesus into your child's life from the beginning?

_____

_____

_____

_____

_____

_____

_____

_____

_____

Can you think of a time during this week when you had fears regarding your child's place in the world? How did God help you overcome those fears?

_____

_____

_____

_____

_____

_____

_____

I know my child has a future to serve you, God. Please help me know how to guide them the right way. (Continue your prayer here.)

_____

_____

_____

_____

_____

_____

_____

Cravings

> *O God, You are my God; earnestly I seek You;*
> *my soul thirsts for You; my flesh faints for You, as*
> *in a dry and weary land where there is no water.*

PSALM 63:1 (NIV)

I'm sure you've had cravings for things you never thought you'd like because of your pregnancy. I remember my go-to drinks, snacks, and sweets, but once I wasn't pregnant anymore, those items really didn't hit the same. I wondered, "What is the big deal with these things, and why do I want them so bad?" Cravings are your body's intense plea for something, and it feels like you really won't survive if you can't get those french fries or that bag of sour candy. The particular food tastes so good once you have it because the desperate yearning for it is finally satisfied.

In the same way, it seems like we crave God only when we're desperate for His presence. Have you ever found yourself crying out for an answer because you just didn't know how you were going to find a new home in time for your growing family, or you just received potentially bad news from your doctor?

Jesus loves to hear from us, and there's a reason we crave Him. He is the source of our strength, our peace, our joy . . . the list goes on and on. If you ever find yourself craving those things, then consider that it's your spirit's way of sending you a craving for more time with Him. Your pregnancy may send you into many ups and downs, but God always provides stability if you allow Him to.

Write down some ways that your relationship with God has helped you in your pregnancy, especially in the unpredictable ups and downs.

_____

_____

_____

_____

_____

_____

_____

_____

_____

When do you find yourself craving time with God the most?

_____

_____

_____

_____

_____

_____

_____

_____

_____

When did praying to God help alleviate your feelings of anxiousness, fear, stress, etc.? Jot down this memory.

_____

_____

_____

_____

_____

_____

_____

_____

God, please help me be more intentional about spending time with You each day. (Continue your prayer here.)

_____

_____

_____

_____

_____

_____

_____

_____

The Wisdom to Obey

> *"Therefore everyone who hears these words of Mine and puts them into practice is like a wise man who built his house on the rock."*
>
> MATTHEW 7:24 (NIV)

As soon as you see that positive pregnancy test, it seems as though time goes into warp speed. Before you know it, you're walking into your first prenatal appointment, where you'll get a list of dos and don'ts and go over your new health regimen. I don't know about you, but it felt like a mountain of work was ahead of me with my first pregnancy. Before then, I not only had no idea how many things I would have to be aware of, but I also didn't realize the high volume of appointments I'd be going to month after month. I remember feeling like "Geez, everything I do revolves around this baby. What about *me*?"

Sometimes rules can make you feel very limited in your options and drain the joy out of such a blessed time in your life. Similar to how Jesus reminds us that it is wise to put His words into action, it's also prudent for you to put into practice the things you're advised to do during your pregnancy. It's not that Jesus wants to rain on your parade; every bit of advice and warning He gives is for your own good.

Perspective is everything. If you understand that the new guidelines for your life, such as changing your diet and avoiding certain activities, are there only to help you and your unborn child be healthy, then you can have a deeper joy in following through with them. By taking care of yourself physically and spiritually during this time, you're setting yourself up for great success in both areas.

13

Is there anything you've learned during your first trimester about the care of your baby and yourself that really took you by surprise?

_____

_____

_____

_____

_____

_____

_____

In a time of "don't do this or that," what are some things you're still able to do while pregnant that you really enjoy?

_____

_____

_____

_____

_____

_____

_____

What were your thoughts and emotions during your first prenatal appointment? Be as detailed as you'd like (this will be fun to look back on).

_____

_____

_____

_____

_____

_____

_____

_____

God, please help me be diligent in taking care of myself by using wisdom during this pregnancy and not forgetting to keep my relationship with You a priority as well. (Continue your prayer here.)

_____

_____

_____

_____

_____

_____

_____

Stop Worry in Its Tracks

> *Can any one of you by worrying add
> a single hour to your life?*
>
> **MATTHEW 6:27 (NIV)**

Your first trimester is known to come with a dark, ominous cloud because you hear stories of what can go wrong in those first few weeks. It's even recommended not to announce your pregnancy yet because anything can happen and you don't want to go through a loss publicly.

Even though my miscarriage was painful, one of the best things I ever did was share my experience on social media. The amount of support I received and was eventually able to give to others who had gone through the same thing took the sting out of such a heavy time in my life. What helped me resist the negative ideas that came up every once in a while after I conceived again was the Word of God. Every day, I spoke scriptures over my unborn child and myself to combat my anxiety so that peace would be the loudest voice.

I kept reminding myself, "What if I spend this whole pregnancy stressed out, only to end up with a healthy kid? What a waste of time that would be!" I trusted that God could and would bless me with a healthy baby, and I was determined to celebrate the life inside of me. As the Bible reminds us, worry adds absolutely nothing to our lives.

You might have gone through unexpected situations in the past when it comes to having a child, but God is by your side every step of the way, and He will not leave you to face anything alone.

What are some ways you can combat anxiety and instead turn it to trust in God?

_____

_____

_____

_____

_____

_____

_____

_____

Write down a time in your first trimester when you felt worried or overwhelmed. How did you get past those emotions?

_____

_____

_____

_____

_____

_____

_____

_____

_____

What activities have you engaged in during your first trimester to get excited about your pregnancy and take your mind off negative thoughts?

_____

_____

_____

_____

_____

_____

_____

_____

Lord, I choose to trust You instead of worry, but I need Your help letting go of fear. (Continue your prayer here.)

_____

_____

_____

_____

_____

_____

_____

_____

Having Hope in the Right Thing

> *For in this hope we were saved. But hope that is seen is no hope at all. Who hopes for what they already have? But if we hope for what we do not yet have, we wait for it patiently.*
>
> ROMANS 8:24–25 (NIV)

People often put their hope in only what they believe is a sure thing. It's often advised not to count your chickens before they hatch. There's even a negative connotation to the phrase "getting your hopes up." As Christians, we put our hope and trust in Jesus Christ. That's what sets us apart in how we live and view things, like planning for the future.

Hope permeates the teachings in the Bible, and each person God called to do something courageous had to keep their faith strong. Expectant women hope they have a pregnancy with no negative symptoms and that labor goes according to their plan. New mothers hope their newborns will sleep through the night. We always have to leave room for God to be involved in this process because things might not always go the way we think they will.

Placing hope in your own abilities can lead to anxiety or stress because you weren't meant to complete this process without His divine presence. We should hope in Him that everything will be okay regardless of the journey. We should hope in Him that He will help us through the highs and lows. We may not see how everything is going to work out, but if we did, then we wouldn't need hope. Keep your hope in the right place, and that's with God alone.

What are some things you've hoped for during your pregnancy that led to disappointment? It's okay to be honest with God about this.

_____

_____

_____

_____

_____

_____

_____

_____

How have you seen God move in unexpected ways to bless you during your pregnancy?

_____

_____

_____

_____

_____

_____

_____

_____

Describe a time when you almost gave up hope in something this past month, but God still came through.

_____

_____

_____

_____

_____

_____

_____

_____

Father, please help me place my hope in You always, instead of in myself or others. (Continue your prayer here.)

_____

_____

_____

_____

_____

_____

_____

_____

Setting a Peaceful Atmosphere

> *For in this hope we were saved. But hope that is seen is no hope at all. Who hopes for what they already have? But if we hope for what we do not yet have, we wait for it patiently.*
>
> **ROMANS 8:24-25 (NIV)**

L ast week I reminded you why it's important to keep your hope in God and His promise to be with you and see you through every high and low. This week I want to highlight the very last word in the passage we visited last week: "patiently." Ephesians 4:2 says, "Be completely humble and gentle; be patient, bearing with one another in love."

As you're waiting patiently for good news regarding your last doctor's appointment, for the nursery furniture to be delivered, and for that stubborn sciatic pain to end for good, remember to be mindful of how you interact with others. Your hormones are most likely taking you on a roller coaster, but it's imperative that you maintain a gentle temperament so that you allow for a steady and peaceful environment for you and your baby.

Jesus came in human form and experienced every emotion we could possibly go through, but something He did to cope with that was go away by Himself from time to time to communicate with the Father. We can handle only so much, and God understands our fragility, so don't feel bad if you need a time-out to cool down. Make quiet time with God a priority so that you can build up again when you're running extremely low on energy or finding it hard to be patient.

Can you think of what things trigger your mood swings and how you can try to avoid those triggers?

_____

_____

_____

_____

_____

_____

_____

What are some ways you can be better at interacting with others or keeping a calm and peaceful temperament?

_____

_____

_____

_____

_____

_____

_____

_____

Was there a time recently when you were able to turn your day around by having a better outlook and choosing to be patient?

_____

_____

_____

_____

_____

_____

_____

God, when I can feel my emotions getting out of control, please help me be peaceful instead. (Continue your prayer here.)

_____

_____

_____

_____

_____

_____

_____

_____

Can You Tame the Tongue?

> *The tongue has the power of life and death,*
> *and those who love it will eat its fruit.*
>
> **PROVERBS 18:21 (NIV)**

In the Amplified Bible Classic Edition (AMPC) translation, this Proverbs scripture states: "Death and life are in the power of the tongue, and those who love it *and* indulge it will eat its fruit *and* bear the consequences of their words." This reading reminds me of a bad habit I developed in my first pregnancy. Between feeling tired and so overwhelmed by becoming a first-time mom, I noticed my conversational "filter" was completely gone, and harsh words I never used to say left my lips before I had the chance to stop them.

Pregnant women should get a free pass for things like this, right? Not according to the Bible. Luke 6:45 says, "A good man brings good things out of the good stored up in his heart, and an evil man brings evil things out of the evil stored up in his heart. For the mouth speaks what the heart is full of." I realized there was a root cause of the painful words I spoke, and it was unhealed hurts of my own. If you need to deal with some wounds in your heart that you haven't addressed yet, then you're not alone.

Wise words in James 1:19 tell us, "My dear brothers and sisters, take note of this: Everyone should be quick to listen, slow to speak, and slow to become angry." I had to allow God to start working on me.

Instead of letting words bubble up without submitting them to Christ first, I would pause and ask myself, "Is this going to be hurtful? Am I being defensive? Will this offend the other person?" If you can't seem to take control of your words or find that filter you had prepregnancy, then you may need to work on your heart. Now is a great time to start your healing.

What are some things you can do when you feel your tone getting harsh or you can't seem to respond in loving ways?

_____

_____

_____

_____

_____

_____

_____

Are you discovering any deep wounds that you need God's help with?

_____

_____

_____

_____

_____

_____

_____

_____

Can you think of a time this week when something caused you to react in a way that was hurtful? It's okay that you made this mistake, and you can learn from it.

_____

_____

_____

_____

_____

_____

_____

_____

I'm not always at my best, Lord, but I am trying to live in a way that is pleasing to You. Please help me heal from anything that may be a hidden wound. (Continue your prayer here.)

_____

_____

_____

_____

_____

_____

_____

_____

Pressing Pause

> *He makes me lie down in green pastures,*
> *He leads me beside quiet waters, He refreshes*
> *my soul. He guides me along the right paths*
> *for His name's sake.*
>
> **PSALM 23:2-3 (NIV)**

All of the fetus's major organs and systems form during your first trimester, and that's why you feel like you can barely keep your eyes open. Brushing your teeth or taking a shower might leave you huffing and puffing like you've just finished a marathon. The road to motherhood is filled with moments that take your breath away, but most are good: the first time you see your baby's sonogram, the first time you feel a tiny kick, and the first time others can *really* tell you're pregnant (and not just full from that huge portion of pasta).

However, you may feel disappointment over not being able to fully enjoy your pregnancy due to the numerous bathroom breaks and aversions to what used to be your favorite foods. It's hard to take care of your to-do lists and schedule appointments when your life is interrupted by six daytime naps.

Fully surrendering yourself to this new season of life is the way to find the good in these changes. Get used to things being a little different and taking longer. The beauty of developing a new life inside of you is that you don't have to feel guilty for taking advantage of God's rest.

Scripture says that He leads us beside quiet waters and refreshes our soul. This goes for those nine months of pregnancy as well. The next time you're feeling bone tired, remember that your little one depends on your ability to pause when you need to. This experience is perfectly normal, and this, too, shall pass.

Have there been times when you found it hard to give in to the rest you need?

_____

_____

_____

_____

_____

_____

_____

_____

Are there any activities you can forgo during this season of your life so that you have more time to rest?

_____

_____

_____

_____

_____

_____

_____

_____

_____

Write about some of the funniest moments when you found yourself nodding off in the middle of trying to get something done.

_____

_____

_____

_____

_____

_____

_____

_____

Please give me strength to make time for myself each day and to take advantage of Your rest, God. (Continue your prayer here.)

_____

_____

_____

_____

_____

_____

_____

_____

Revisit That To-Do List

> *In their hearts humans plan their course,*
> *but the Lord establishes their steps.*
>
> **PROVERBS 16:9 (NIV)**

There's an old Yiddish saying, "Man plans, and God laughs." Looking back on my life, so many things haven't gone as I hoped or imagined. I'd love to have an idea of what's up next in my future, but my life has not been—and most likely never will be—laid out according to a predictable plan.

I'm sure you can relate. Perhaps you had grand plans to complete your nursery during your second trimester—while you still have energy—only to have your baby's furniture delivery delayed by two months. Maybe your baby shower was supposed to be at a certain venue on a specific date, but they suddenly informed you that they mistakenly overbooked.

During this pregnancy, it may be helpful for you to revisit your to-do list with two versions: "Must-haves" and "Would be nice." As long as your top priorities are accomplished (and you keep them to a minimum), you'll give room for God to work and get rid of a lot of unnecessary stress.

We may plan a course, but ultimately it's God who knows what's best for us. You might be surprised by how well everything works out with things that are beyond your control. That furniture delay could make room for a major sale that you didn't expect to take advantage of. Your new baby shower date might allow your best friend from out of town, who was previously unavailable, to attend.

What are some things you feel must be accomplished
this week?

_____

_____

_____

_____

_____

_____

_____

_____

What are some plans that you could be more flexible with
this week?

_____

_____

_____

_____

_____

_____

_____

_____

Was there a time during this pregnancy when your plans fell through and made room for a major blessing from God?

_____

_____

_____

_____

_____

_____

_____

_____

God, please help me be flexible with my plans when things come up that are unexpected. (Continue your prayer here.)

_____

_____

_____

_____

_____

_____

_____

_____

It's Okay to Miss "Her"

> *How precious to me are Your thoughts,*
> *God! How vast is the sum of them!*
>
> **PSALM 139:17 (NIV)**

I was on social media the other day and saw a pregnant woman reminiscing about her prepregnant self with a caption that included the words "I miss her." Pregnancy is one of the most beautiful seasons in a woman's life, so why is it that many pregnant women don't feel beautiful? Imagine standing in front of a mirror and the reflection staring back at you looks like a stranger. I bet you don't have to imagine because you're most likely living it, right?

Your body may be changing, and so is your world and how you move within it. For example, the freedom to get up and go without wondering if the car ride will make you nauseous or if your knees will give out on you at the grocery store are experiences you had with your prepregnant life. In the same way, looking at your pregnancy announcement pictures may bring back bittersweet memories of an aching back or how challenging it was to get dressed in the morning because of swollen feet and ankles.

No matter what negative thoughts or feelings you have about your body right now, God's thoughts are always positive toward you, and He knows the wonderful internal and external changes you're experiencing right now will forever be a part of you.

It's important to be intentional about building ourselves up, telling ourselves what a good job we're doing, and reminding ourselves what a blessing this season is to grow in exponential ways. You're not losing yourself in motherhood—you're gaining a new part of yourself.

If you feel unhappy, then it might be helpful to write down some things you look forward to doing after pregnancy.

_____

_____

_____

_____

_____

_____

_____

How do you think you've changed for the better while pregnant?

_____

_____

_____

_____

_____

_____

_____

_____

List some things that have happened this past month that made you happy to be pregnant.

_____

_____

_____

_____

_____

_____

_____

_____

Lord, I know you always see me as beautiful and Your thoughts toward me are precious. Help me see myself the same way You do. (Continue your prayer here.)

_____

_____

_____

_____

_____

_____

_____

_____

"Why Don't I Look Like Them?"

> *A heart at peace gives life to the body,*
> *but envy rots the bones.*
>
> **PROVERBS 14:30 (NIV)**

An innocent online search for maternity outfit ideas will alert the algorithm to flood your screen with the cutest photos of pregnant women you've ever seen. Speaking from experience, I encourage you to resist the urge to pick yourself apart. Most likely you'll end up scrolling through your social media feed and feeling jealous of other pregnant women. "Her belly is so much smaller than mine." "Look at how gorgeous and smooth her skin is." "I just can't seem to get myself together these days."

Instead, focus on the things you love about your pregnant self. Something I loved about being pregnant was that it drastically reduced my desire to please people. It helped me stand up for myself because I no longer had the energy to pretend that people's hurtful actions or words did not bother me.

There's a reason scripture says that peace gives life and envy rots the bones. So many of our thoughts manifest into the way we feel. Think about it: Have you ever felt sick to your stomach or had a pounding headache because of stress? Take care of your emotional well-being and your body right now by refusing to fall into a comparison trap.

If you often spiral into sadness while on social media, then you might want to limit how much you are online. I know, I know . . . it's hard because most of your time might be spent on the couch or in bed these days, but try to find other things to do.

Are there any physical traits you love about your pregnant self? List them here.

_____

_____

_____

_____

_____

_____

_____

How has pregnancy transformed your character in a positive way?

_____

_____

_____

_____

_____

_____

_____

_____

What are some of the fun and productive things you've been able to do this past month instead of scrolling online?

_____

_____

_____

_____

_____

_____

_____

_____

Father, when I have an urge to compare myself with other women, please help me redirect my thoughts to be more uplifting. (Continue your prayer here.)

_____

_____

_____

_____

_____

_____

_____

Have You Talked to God About It?

> *Do not be anxious about anything, but in every situation, by prayer and petition, with thanksgiving, present your requests to God. And the peace of God, which transcends all understanding, will guard your hearts and your minds in Christ Jesus.*
>
> **PHILIPPIANS 4:6–7 (NIV)**

One of the "fun" symptoms that often comes up for pregnant women in their second and/or third trimester is insomnia. By "fun" I mean you spend all night tossing and turning because you can't get comfortable, or your bladder will wake you up at the worst possible time. Once you're up, shutting your brain off is hard.

While you're staring at the ceiling, it's common to start thinking of the things that trigger anxiety. Maybe you've been dealing with drama among your friend group. Perhaps at your last doctor visit, your blood pressure was a bit high. None of these things help you relax. Scripture reminds us that we aren't supposed to be anxious, so how do you combat a normal human emotion like that? With prayer. With thanksgiving. By talking to God about it.

God knows we as humans will go through seasons and circumstances that shake our peace. Instead of trying to figure out everything yourself, offer God the space to be in this with you. He wants you to be covered in His peace so that He can guard your heart. By having consistent conversations with Him, you'll find more rest in your heart despite those sleepless nights and sometimes tiring days.

Write down a few things you're thankful for currently.

_____

_____

_____

_____

_____

_____

_____

_____

If you are concerned about anything in your life, then how have you been praying about those concerns?

_____

_____

_____

_____

_____

_____

_____

_____

_____

_____

What is one major way you've felt God's presence this week when worries came up?

_____

_____

_____

_____

_____

_____

_____

So much is out of my control, but I know nothing is a surprise to You. Lord, please remind me to run to You before I get over-whelmed. (Continue your prayer here.)

_____

_____

_____

_____

_____

_____

_____

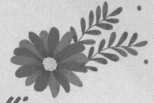

Ignore the Headlines

> *So do not fear, for I am with you; do not*
> *be dismayed, for I am your God. I will strengthen*
> *you and help you; I will uphold you with*
> *My righteous right hand.*

ISAIAH 41:10 (NIV)

Turn on any news channel or open up a newspaper and you'll see stories that will grip you with fear. Actually, no. *Don't* do that, although it's nearly impossible to get away from the headlines even when running simple errands (you can thank the person who came up with the idea to install TVs at gas pumps). Perhaps you were fine dealing with this before having kids, but most longtime mothers and even new moms can't help but imagine the worst for our children when we see the Top 10 most popular news stories from around the globe.

Keeping our eyes on what the world is up to robs us of the day-to-day joys we could be reveling in. It also causes us to deny the power of our prayers. The Bible says in James 5:16, "The prayer of a righteous person is powerful and effective." Pray instead of worry. Pray instead of doubting. You're learning one of the greatest lessons about your role as a mother, which is to fall on your knees instead of falling into the media trap.

I'm giving you an assignment today, and it's simple: Ignore the headlines. Easier said than done, but you'll thank me later. Instead of turning on the evening news, find a sermon on YouTube.

It's a great way to keep God's righteousness at the forefront of your mind. In addition to that, filling your home with praise and worship music will remind you of how God is always there to help you.

How can you avoid being reeled in to news stories that fill you with fear?

_____

_____

_____

_____

_____

_____

_____

Write down some ways you can purposely inject good news into your day-to-day life. (For example, you can find sermons online, listen to praise and worship at work, ask friends for prayer, etc.)

_____

_____

_____

_____

_____

_____

_____

Write down some good news that happened to you personally in your pregnancy this past week.

_____

_____

_____

_____

_____

_____

_____

_____

Lord, there is always bad news that I could focus on, but please help me pay attention to the good that You're doing in my life instead. (Continue your prayer here.)

_____

_____

_____

_____

_____

_____

_____

_____

Motherhood Is . . .

> *For we are God's handiwork, created in*
> *Christ Jesus to do good works, which*
> *God prepared in advance for us to do.*

EPHESIANS 2:10 (NIV)

Close your eyes and think about what motherhood means to you. Once you're finished, open your eyes and keep reading. Maybe your thoughts revolved around taking good care of your children or being a good mom. Interestingly, the Oxford English Dictionary defines motherhood as the state of being a mother. That's it.

Oftentimes we tend to overthink our role as moms. Although motherhood is a grand blessing, who you are as a mother is just an extension of who you are as a person. I've seen many women lose themselves in motherhood because the tasks become their identity. A mom cooks. A mom cleans. A mom takes care of her children. Right? Wrong. Those are activities you *do,* but they don't make you a mother.

Having children is what makes you a mother, but how you fill those shoes is up to you. I remember having somewhat of an identity crisis when my first child was born. I was continually thinking, "Who am I, and what do I do with my life now?" It seemed like I had to choose between prioritizing my daughter and prioritizing myself. I didn't know I could do both.

It wasn't until I started engaging in the activities I loved before having a child that I realized how much I missed and needed those outlets. Don't forget who God made you to be. You're still that person, but you have more things to do and more people to love now. Remember to revisit this concept on days when you feel lost in the tasks and chores that come with taking care of a new little human.

What are some activities that make you come alive, and how can you continue to incorporate those things as a mother?

_____

_____

_____

_____

_____

_____

_____

What are some things that have been hard to give up during your pregnancy and make you miss your old self?

_____

_____

_____

_____

_____

_____

_____

_____

Think of a time this past month when you really enjoyed yourself and felt like "you" again, even while pregnant.

_____

_____

_____

_____

_____

_____

_____

Lord, when I get lost in my role as a mother, please help me remember who I am at my core. (Continue your prayer here.)

_____

_____

_____

_____

_____

_____

_____

_____

He Is Worthy

> *Praise the Lord. Praise God in His sanctuary; praise Him in His mighty heavens. Praise Him for His acts of power; praise Him for His surpassing greatness. Praise Him with the sounding of the trumpet, praise Him with the harp and lyre, praise Him with timbrel and dancing, praise Him with the strings and pipe, praise Him with the clash of cymbals, praise Him with resounding cymbals. Let everything that has breath praise the Lord. Praise the Lord.*
>
> **PSALM 150:1-6 (NIV)**

Usually, the idea of praising God inspires Christians to play the latest popular worship song. Though music is a *form* of praise, the act of praise means to express approval or admiration. Scripture tells us to praise Him for His power and greatness.

There are so many things He's done that can take your breath away, like creating new life out of thin air. During both of my pregnancies, I couldn't tell you how many times I said to myself, "I can't believe there's a whole human inside of me!" Feeling your baby's first kick or seeing their image at your first ultrasound appointment can leave you speechless and remind you of how much reverence you have for God.

We're told over and over in the Bible how much our Father loves us and how precious we are to Him, and it's important that we remember to reciprocate that love to Him as well. We often use prayer to ask for things, but the next time you're talking to God, remind Him of all the reasons you love and adore Him.

When you spend quality time with God, what are some ways you can add more elements of praise into your conversations with Him?

_____

_____

_____

_____

_____

_____

_____

How have the different stages of your pregnancy impacted the deepness of your relationship with Jesus?

_____

_____

_____

_____

_____

_____

_____

_____

What were your emotions the first time you felt your baby kick or the first time you saw them at an ultrasound appointment?

_____

_____

_____

_____

_____

_____

_____

_____

God, you are worthy of all praise. Thank you for the powerful and great things You do for me and my baby. (Continue your prayer here.)

_____

_____

_____

_____

_____

_____

_____

_____

Even Nature Sings

> *The meadows are covered with flocks*
> *and the valleys are mantled with grain;*
> *they shout for joy and sing.*
>
> **PSALM 65:13 (NIV)**

Have you ever been so excited about good news that it feels like everything around you comes to life? Driving down the coast of Southern California, I've seen the water sparkle like it is dancing in the waves. Winding through the mountains of North Carolina, I've heard the dewy leaves rustling to create a gentle lullaby as the sun sets. Walking on the beach in Hawaii with my husband, I could literally feel romance in the humid breeze.

When I first read David's words in Psalm 65—meadows and valleys breaking into song—it sounded like a fairy tale my six-year-old would love. But when I began digging deeper, it was easy to understand David's excitement about what God was doing in his life, the lives of those around him, and even in the land he lived in.

Feeling a deep gratitude opens up your mind to the vast nature of God. The next time you sit before Him, I encourage you to go outside and enjoy the work of His hands. Talk to Him about the joy you feel thinking about the baby growing inside of you and how much you appreciate what He's doing in the lives of your loved ones as well.

God put so much detail into creating a beautiful world for us to dwell in, and it's beneficial for us to be still and take it all in. As the Creator who pays attention to every detail, it's no wonder even the flowers smile in bloom because of the heavenly rain He sends down from above.

Does being outside in nature help you feel closer to God?

_____

_____

_____

_____

_____

_____

_____

_____

When was the last time you really spoke to God and
listed every blessing He's given you during this trimester?
If it's been awhile, then you can start by listing some
things here.

_____

_____

_____

_____

_____

_____

_____

_____

_____

Write about a time this trimester when you received such good news about your baby on the way that it felt like everyone and everything was celebrating with you.

_____

_____

_____

_____

_____

_____

_____

I can't put into words how great Your works are, Father. I'm so excited about my baby, and I thank You for every new milestone I'm experiencing as my baby grows. (Continue your prayer here.)

_____

_____

_____

_____

_____

_____

_____

Trust Fall

> *But blessed is the one who trusts in the Lord,*
> *whose confidence is in Him.*
>
> **JEREMIAH 17:7 (NIV)**

My son is currently learning to walk by holding on to furniture to stabilize him as he takes steps around the house. Even though he stumbles, we're usually an arm's length away, ready to catch him and put him back on his feet. When I think of his attempts at being upright, it reminds me of the "trust fall" technique you've probably witnessed as a team-building exercise. One person falls back with their eyes closed as another person stands behind them ready to catch their weight.

I wish I could say that I've always had confidence in God to catch me. However, I spent the majority of my life doing everything I could not to fail because I wasn't sure what would happen if I didn't have a tight grip on life. I left very little room for the possibility of failure, and it really impeded my growth as a person and hindered what I was capable of doing with my future.

You might feel like people expect you to have everything under control during this pregnancy. More often than not, they're asking about your cravings, your doctor appointments, and when your baby shower is instead of genuinely asking if there's anything you need or if you have enough emotional support.

Even if you do have people coming over to build nursery furniture or help you move, don't forget to bring up the way your community can offer support by praying for you. Despite having others lend a hand, remember that your complete trust should be found in Jesus. He's always there to catch you more than anyone else possibly could.

What things are you trusting God for right now? Be as specific or general as you'd like.

_____

_____

_____

_____

_____

_____

_____

_____

Have you had spiritual support from friends or family recently? Whether your answer is yes or no, has that helped you trust God more?

_____

_____

_____

_____

_____

_____

_____

_____

Write down a memory of something that happened this past month that reminded you God has your back.

_____

_____

_____

_____

_____

_____

_____

_____

Father, please help me trust You more with everything I'm facing in my pregnancy. Thank you for the many ways You're there when I need You. (Continue your prayer here.)

_____

_____

_____

_____

_____

_____

_____

_____

Clueless

> *In my distress I called to the Lord; I cried to my God for help. From His temple He heard my voice; my cry came before Him, into His ears.*
>
> **PSALM 18:6 (NIV)**

Not too long ago, I was checking in on a mom who had just had a baby. Though this was her third child, she mentioned how hard the first several weeks had been because her newborn was crying for most of the day and night with no known cause. Colic had never happened with her other two daughters. Even after checking with the pediatrician, they found nothing wrong and she was assured that some babies just cry uncontrollably, and there wasn't much she could do about it. This mother felt completely helpless and clueless.

One late night she was startled awake again by her child's cries. She felt a nudge from the Holy Spirit to look up signs of lactose intolerance in babies. Incessant crying was one of the common symptoms. After switching to a nondairy formula, she could describe her baby as "a completely new kid."

Switching formulas wasn't on her mind at all until she resolved to pray about a remedy that would bring her baby comfort. Not all treatments for your baby have to be divinely inspired, but this is a reminder that the power of prayer is real, and your Father is available to you at any time.

If you are looking for a solution to something that's been very difficult for you recently, then keep in mind to incorporate prayer into any and every challenge you face. God is always ready and willing to listen.

If you haven't been encouraged to pray lately, then take the time to write down a few things you can bring up to God now.

_____

_____

_____

_____

_____

_____

_____

In addition to the medical support you already have, what are some ways you can trust God to give you personal advice when you need it?

_____

_____

_____

_____

_____

_____

_____

_____

Describe a moment from the past month when you felt like you got an answer directly from heaven about a problem you were dealing with.

_____

_____

_____

_____

_____

_____

_____

God, you know what challenges I'm facing in my pregnancy right now. Please give me Your divine advice on how to deal with them. (Continue your prayer here.)

_____

_____

_____

_____

_____

_____

_____

_____

Where You'll Find Joy

> *You make known to me the path of life;*
> *you will fill me with joy in your presence,*
> *with eternal pleasures at your right hand.*
>
> **PSALM 16:11 (NIV)**

Joy has become a dangling carrot in front of the faces of many people—even expectant mothers—because most people find joy in things that don't last. You may have thought, "I'll be happy when I'm pregnant. I'll be happy when I see that first sonogram. I'll be happy when I'm not so tired. I'll be happy when I'm finally *not* pregnant. I'll be happy when I meet my baby. I'll be happy when . . ." However, joy is a choice, and it comes from being close to God.

For some of you, this pregnancy has been years in the making. You may be confused as to why you're not more content with the child you've been praying for, after waiting for so long to become a mother.

Whenever we allow outside circumstances to dictate how we feel, we miss out on the steady flow of happiness that can come only from Jesus. Understanding that Jesus is the ultimate prize and gift can change our entire outlook on life and give us that inexpressible and glorious joy mentioned in 1 Peter 1:8: "Though you have not seen Him, you love Him; and even though you do not see Him now, you believe in Him and are filled with an inexpressible and glorious joy." You can choose now to make a commitment to finding joy where it resides instead of chasing it where it doesn't exist.

Do you have a pattern of mostly finding joy in things that don't last? Why or why not?

_____

_____

_____

_____

_____

_____

_____

What are some ways you can find joy in your walk with God?

_____

_____

_____

_____

_____

_____

_____

_____

Write down a few memories of how you felt when you spent more time with God. What about when you spent less time with God?

_____

_____

_____

_____

_____

_____

_____

_____

Lord, I understand that having joy is a choice. Please help me keep You as my focus when I'm feeling discontent. (Continue your prayer here.)

_____

_____

_____

_____

_____

_____

_____

Is This God's Plan?

> *And we know that in all things God works for the good of those who love Him, who have been called according to His purpose.*
>
> **ROMANS 8:28 (NIV)**

A mom I follow on social media was sharing how she was trying not to feel like she was robbed of her full pregnancy experience in the year 2020. Everyone across the globe was affected by a pandemic, and the usual concerns of being with child coupled with a virus that ravaged the world left many pregnant women (including myself) with a huge emotional burden.

Pandemic or not, there are most likely things you've experienced that have come out of left field and had you questioning if this was God's plan. One thing is for sure: No matter what comes your way, God can make use of it. It doesn't mean He caused it, because we do live in a world with death, disease, and sin. Despite this, His children are always on His mind.

God sees you and understands your disappointment when things don't go according to your hopes or desires. It's true that God will finish every good thing He started in your life. According to Philippians 1:6, "He who began a good work in You will carry it on to completion until the day of Christ Jesus." As long as you give Him room to do so, He will work everything out in your favor. If your story isn't good, then it's not over. If you're in the middle of a storm, then hold tight because His help is on the way.

Are there any things that are beyond your control that have been hard to cope with during your pregnancy?

_____

_____

_____

_____

_____

_____

_____

_____

How do world events affect your faith for good or bad?

_____

_____

_____

_____

_____

_____

_____

_____

_____

_____

This past month, how have you seen God turn something into a positive that started out being negative?

_____

_____

_____

_____

_____

_____

_____

God, I've had some disappointments that I want to bring before You today. Please help me heal the hurt that came along with those. (Continue your prayer here.)

_____

_____

_____

_____

_____

_____

_____

_____

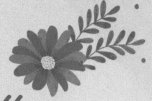

WEEK 23

Preparing Your Home

> *My people will live in peaceful dwelling places,*
> *in secure homes, in undisturbed places of rest.*
>
> **ISAIAH 32:18 (NIV)**

When a mom thinks of preparing her home for a baby, the idea of nesting is what usually comes to mind. She declutters. She cleans the crevices that haven't been swept in a while. She gets all the onesies washed, folded, and put away. These tasks are important, and you'll be so glad you've completed them before you're too tired and breathless to do much more. However, it's just as important to prepare the right tone for your home's atmosphere.

I want you to look forward to the upcoming days, weeks, and months with your new baby by doing what it takes to build your spiritual nest now. While you still have a chance, figure out how you can take time with God each day. Be realistic! You can begin by turning on praise and worship music and praying over your family for five minutes.

Also, now is a good time to think about how many visitors you'll want to have and who they'll be. You probably have a good gauge on who will actually be helpful, who will just want to hold the baby, and who might overstay their welcome. It's also important to think about doing things that help you feel like yourself.

How can you incorporate your favorite show, get in a solid 30-minute bath, or dig in to your love for cooking–even if it's once a week? Deciding on these things in advance is a great way to prepare your home to be a peaceful refuge for you and the little one on the way.

67

What are some ways you can give God time each day, starting even now?

_____

_____

_____

_____

_____

_____

_____

What are some of the things that make you feel like yourself that you can incorporate once a week after the baby arrives?

_____

_____

_____

_____

_____

_____

_____

_____

Describe a time recently when you felt at peace in your home. What caused that?

_____

_____

_____

_____

_____

_____

_____

_____

God, I don't even know where to begin when it comes to pre-paring my home emotionally and spiritually. Please guide me in this. (Continue your prayer here.)

_____

_____

_____

_____

_____

_____

_____

_____

Letting Go

> But the fruit of the Spirit is love, joy, peace,
> forbearance, kindness, goodness, faithfulness,
> gentleness, and self-control. Against such
> things there is no law.
>
> **GALATIANS 5:22-23 (NIV)**

They say the newborn period of your first child's life is one of the hardest times a mom will go through. That was my experience, and I thought that was normal because online articles promised it would be. It wasn't until I met a few moms who reminisced fondly of those sleepless nights and newborn coos that I discovered this wasn't the case for all.

Once when I was at a baby shower, a woman talked about being waited on hand and foot for her first month as a mom. "You better make this the best experience for me if you want me to have any more kids," she recalled telling her family and friends, who agreed. There was a pattern here; a solid support system.

It takes a village to raise a child, but there isn't enough emphasis on having the *right* individuals in that village. Surrounding yourself with people doesn't always get rid of the woes of life after labor and delivery. My experience with newborn number two was drastically different from my first. The main change? I cut out people, habits, and circumstances that were toxic to my well-being. It made a world of difference, and that can be the case for you as well.

I recommend doing a spiritual and emotional inventory check for your life. In Galatians, we read what God considers the fruit of the Spirit. If there are people in your life or even characteristics within yourself that don't line up with that, then it's time to start "cleaning house."

Which people in your life do you consider a healthy support system?

_____

_____

_____

_____

_____

_____

_____

_____

Which people in your life do you consider unsupportive?

_____

_____

_____

_____

_____

_____

_____

_____

Are there times when you felt very supported or highly dismissed during your pregnancy? What specifically brought about those feelings?

_____

_____

_____

_____

_____

_____

_____

God, please help me draw closer to those I need in my life and cut out those who should be removed. (Continue your prayer here.)

_____

_____

_____

_____

_____

_____

_____

_____

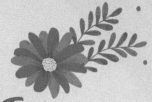

Forgiveness Is Free

> *Be kind and compassionate to one another,*
> *forgiving each other, just as in Christ*
> *God forgave you.*
>
> **EPHESIANS 4:32 (NIV)**

I've heard countless stories from other mothers about how becoming a parent allowed them to see their own parents with more compassion and grace. When you're a child, your caretaker is somewhat of a superhero to you. You assume they know everything and can accomplish anything, so when that person falls short, it's hard not to carry that disappointment from childhood well into adulthood. However, *all* people fail, and it's only because of Jesus Christ that God redeems us to become whole and forgiven.

True forgiveness from God means that He forgets our wrongdoings and is faithful to see us as His precious children. He also calls us to do the same for those who have wronged us. Letting go is especially important for those of you who have dealt with trauma in the past. Forgiveness doesn't cost us anything, but it doesn't mean that choosing to move on will be easy.

You don't have to live in an anxious state of mind hoping you won't make the same mistakes as a mother that your caretakers made with you. The amazing thing about God's grace is that it comes with the power to transform you from the inside out.

If you walk away from the bitterness you may be holding on to or even the regret of your past downfalls, then you can see this chapter in your life as a clean slate and offer yourself to God as a vessel that is turning over a new leaf for the next generations.

What are some things you need to forgive yourself for?

_____

_____

_____

_____

_____

_____

_____

Who are some people you need to forgive in order to be released from the pain you might be feeling?

_____

_____

_____

_____

_____

_____

_____

_____

Can you think of a time in this past week when you were able to forgive someone for a mistake they made?

_____

_____

_____

_____

_____

_____

_____

Father, my heart is hurting from wounds caused in my past. Please heal my heart so that I can completely move on from this pain. (Continue your prayer here.)

_____

_____

_____

_____

_____

_____

_____

_____

Temporary Pain

> *I consider that our present sufferings*
> *are not worth comparing with the glory*
> *that will be revealed in us.*
>
> **ROMANS 8:18 (NIV)**

It's true that pregnancy can take a toll on us and feel like forever until we experience the sweet relief of getting our bodies back. You might find yourself counting down the days to your due date. It's normal to shed a few tears when everything makes you nauseous and your back is screaming from walking to and from the kitchen. Whether it's the next season or the next few days, it's hard not to anticipate what's coming up or wish for time to speed up because of the challenges you might be going through emotionally, physically, or mentally as you wait for your baby to arrive.

However, this Romans verse reminds us that all sufferings are not worth comparing with the good that is to come. When you hold your sweet baby in your arms, you won't be thinking about the pain you've gone through. You'll be so happy for this new beginning and the good times ahead.

Sure, you may remember the nausea during your first trimester or the discomfort of your third trimester and think, "I'm never doing this again." Perhaps you're one of the mamas who has had children before and decided that the pain was worth it to give it another round. No matter what is weighing heavy on you, understand that it's temporary.

Keep your mind on what is to come and do your best to enjoy the time that you have while your baby is in the womb. Try to enjoy the preparation process with a thankful heart. It might be hard for you, but it will not last forever. That's worth rejoicing over!

What are some of the present sufferings you've been dealing with this week?

_____

_____

_____

_____

_____

_____

_____

_____

What are some of the future things you're looking forward to once the baby is here?

_____

_____

_____

_____

_____

_____

_____

_____

Are there any hardships you can look back on throughout your pregnancy that seemed difficult at the time but that you were able to overcome?

_____

_____

_____

_____

_____

_____

_____

When time seems to pass slowly and the symptoms of my pregnancy are weighing heavily on me, please help me have a thankful heart, Lord. (Continue your prayer here.)

_____

_____

_____

_____

_____

_____

_____

_____

"I Can't Do This Anymore!"

> *I can do all this through Him who gives me strength.*
>
> **PHILIPPIANS 4:13 (NIV)**

When I was traveling to one of my last prenatal appointments, I could feel my stomach churning and I knew what was coming next. While riding passenger side in the carpool lane at 65 miles per hour, I did the only thing I could–reached for a barf bag. I remember crying and screaming, "I can't do this anymore!"

Weeks later, after my baby was making his way down the birth canal and the pain was almost unbearable, I screamed for help as if someone else could deliver the baby for me. Even though I had given birth once before, I was convinced I couldn't do it this time. My midwife and her assistant kept reminding me, "You're the only one who can do this and you're doing great." Someone repeating that I could do this was the main thing that kept me going as I called out to God during intense contractions. I must have worn out His ear with how many times I screamed His name.

Once my son made his slippery way into the world after my final push, I sat in shock that I had actually done it. I was in disbelief for hours that I had completed what felt like an impossible task. We're reminded in the Bible that we can do "all this" through Him who gives us strength. "All this" means "anything."

Whatever doubts you have in your ability to endure this pregnancy, get through labor and delivery, or survive the newborn stage of sleepless nights, remember it's *His* strength flowing through you that will get it done. You don't have to navigate the process alone. How great is that comfort?

Are there any things coming up that you feel you're not capable of handling?

_____

_____

_____

_____

_____

_____

_____

_____

What are some ways you feel weak and need God's help?

_____

_____

_____

_____

_____

_____

_____

_____

_____

Look back on your entire pregnancy and list some things you overcame that you didn't think you would.

_____

_____

_____

_____

_____

_____

_____

_____

God, I don't always feel equipped to handle the circumstances that come with my pregnancy. Please remind me when I'm overwhelmed that I can do anything with You by my side. (Continue your prayer here.)

_____

_____

_____

_____

_____

_____

_____

Together as a Team

*If it is possible, as far as it depends on you,
live at peace with everyone.*

ROMANS 12:18 (NIV)

Welcoming new life is as stressful as it is exciting, so it's no wonder why many couples argue throughout the pregnancy and well into the newborn stage. Perhaps one of you wants to co-sleep with the baby, whereas the other thinks the crib is the best way to go when the baby comes. Maybe one of you thinks you should be asking for more help preparing your home, whereas the other can't stand the idea of having another person come over and be in your personal space. Whatever the topic, you won't always agree with your partner. What do you do in those times when you both are at the end of your rope?

Praying together is a way of hitting a reset button on the day. When tensions rise, it's best to give space for a moment of clarity. You might have noticed that when you're able to take a break or maybe just leave the room for a few minutes, you can de-escalate an argument and significantly cut down on the time you spend debating each other.

Another thing that prayer does is allow God into the situation, shifting your focus back onto Him. If your perspective is to see your partner as someone who's in the way versus your long-term teammate, then you're more likely to take out your frustrations on them.

Whether you have a significant other or maybe a friend or family member walking you through this journey, keep the health of your relationship as a top priority by working together as a team.

When you are tempted to argue as emotions run high, what are some practical ways you can combat that?

_____

_____

_____

_____

_____

_____

_____

_____

Are there any negative habits you have that you can work on now in order to purposefully live at peace?

_____

_____

_____

_____

_____

_____

_____

_____

_____

Describe a time recently when you were able to have a productive conversation instead of it turning into an argument.

_____

_____

_____

_____

_____

_____

_____

_____

God, please help me keep my close relationships healthy. (Continue your prayer here.)

_____

_____

_____

_____

_____

_____

_____

_____

Thanks Be to God

> *Rejoice always, pray continually, give thanks in all circumstances; for this is God's will for you in Christ Jesus.*
>
> **1 THESSALONIANS 5:16-18 (NIV)**

Years ago I was talking to a family member who was struggling with depressing thoughts and trying to get out of an emotional funk. Even though their circumstances weren't related to a pregnancy, it reminded me of a time when I was mentally struggling with the difficult symptoms of my third trimester.

It's hard when you feel like your day begins with a heavy weight. What has helped me in the past is what I offered my family member over the phone. I told them to make a list of 10 things they're thankful for, because when we're focused on what God is doing right, it's harder to think about what's going wrong.

I'd like to offer you the same advice. It's already difficult to keep a smile on our faces without all of the pregnancy hormones sending us into an emotional whirlwind, so take time to focus on the positives for your own good. God has done so much for us, and we cannot forget to praise Him and remind Him how grateful we are for those things.

Sometimes we take for granted that we have the blessing of carrying new life or that we're entering an exciting chapter of motherhood. Let's be children who care to show appreciation instead of complaints.

What are some things you're grateful for today?

_____

_____

_____

_____

_____

_____

_____

How can you be more grateful in your relationship with God overall?

_____

_____

_____

_____

_____

_____

_____

_____

_____

List some things that have happened in your pregnancy recently that you're thankful for.

_____

_____

_____

_____

_____

_____

_____

_____

Lord, I want to take a moment right now not to ask You for anything, but just to thank You for what You're doing in my pregnancy. (Continue your prayer here.)

_____

_____

_____

_____

_____

_____

_____

_____

"Can I Speak to the Manager?"

> *Do to others as you would have them do to you.*
>
> **LUKE 6:31 (NIV)**

Last week I wrote about being thankful to God. We're continuing with the theme of thankfulness, but this time I'd like to put a spotlight on how we treat others. If you've ever been looking for a place to eat, a local nail salon, or even a moving service, then you've probably read the reviews for that business before making your final decision. When people have had bad experiences, they let others know. Fortunately, there are people who give rave reviews because of their positive experiences, too.

When was the last time you made an intentional effort to honor those who are encouraging you through your pregnancy? You can start by expressing your gratitude to your support system or letting the staff at your doctor's office know how much you appreciate them. It can turn their whole day around!

I thought about this when pleasantly grocery shopping one day. I knew it would mean a lot to the staff and management if I complimented them in person. I asked to speak to the manager, and he walked over as if bracing himself for impact. I told him what a great job everyone was doing, and his face lit up. He couldn't stop thanking me for taking the time to say something.

Your mommy brain might have you fixated mostly on self instead of others right now, and that's totally normal. I encourage you to be the voice out there uplifting others by telling them all the good they're doing. It will make the world of difference for them and bless your heart as well.

Are there any people who come to mind that you can offer more kindness?

_____

_____

_____

_____

_____

_____

_____

_____

Write down some ways you can express your gratitude, even if it's complimenting the staff at your prenatal appointments and other places you go.

_____

_____

_____

_____

_____

_____

_____

_____

Can you remember a time this past month when you went out of your way to thank someone? How did that impact your day?

_____

_____

_____

_____

_____

_____

_____

Father, please inspire me in more moments throughout my day to be thankful and kind to others. (Continue your prayer here.)

_____

_____

_____

_____

_____

_____

_____

_____

Is It the Lord's Will?

> Now listen, you who say, "Today or tomorrow
> we will go to this or that city, spend a year
> there, carry on business and make money."
> Why, you do not even know what will happen
> tomorrow. What is your life? You are a mist that
> appears for a little while and then vanishes.
> Instead, you ought to say, "If it is the Lord's will,
> we will live and do this or that."
>
> **JAMES 4:13–15 (NIV)**

There are few things more unpredictable than pregnancy. Even your due date is usually a guesstimate. The unknown that already comes with life is greatly amplified. For some of you, that is simply more than you can handle right now. I've felt that way too many times for me to count. In my ninth month of pregnancy, a wildfire broke out close to my home. The night before, I already smelled a hint of smoke coming through the windows. By early morning, I got an emergency alert on my phone to evacuate our neighborhood.

Before the fire, I had already made plans to do my usual lying around the house between potty breaks because my stomach was getting so heavy at that point. I was sure that my days leading up to giving birth would be uneventful. The Bible reminds us that making long-term plans with our limited knowledge is never guaranteed because it's only He who knows what the future holds.

This doesn't mean you can't make any plans at all; it just proves that those plans will go through only if it is the Lord's will. Diligently seek God daily to help you become more flexible in your pregnancy-related plans so that you aren't completely in shock if you're caught off guard.

How has it made you feel when things were outside of your control during your pregnancy?

_____

_____

_____

_____

_____

_____

_____

_____

Does knowing that God is always there in life's unpredictable moments bring you comfort?

_____

_____

_____

_____

_____

_____

_____

_____

Describe any time within this trimester when something major came up that you didn't expect. How did you deal with it?

_____

_____

_____

_____

_____

_____

_____

God, I have my plans, but I want Your plans for me to prosper in my life. Please help me be more flexible when things don't go how I want them to. (Continue your prayer here.)

_____

_____

_____

_____

_____

_____

_____

_____

Trusting God to Provide

> *Look at the birds of the air; they do not sow or reap or store away in barns, and yet your heavenly Father feeds them. Are you not much more valuable than they?*
>
> **MATTHEW 6:26 (NIV)**

I was talking to a friend on the phone during the tail end of my first pregnancy. She asked how I was doing, and I told her I was trying not to stress out about the things I had left to do and items I still needed to buy before my baby was born. She reassured me that all my baby really needed was their mama and some diapers. I thought that was a kind sentiment, but surely I didn't spend so much time on a registry and a nursery for my daughter to need just diapers.

Here I am years later with two kids, and I now fully agree that there isn't much you're required to have in order to take care of a baby. Their needs are basic, but every store you register with will have 10 categories of baby care and dozens of "must-haves" on their curated list. It's hard not to feel overwhelmed.

Perhaps you're in a small space as a first-time mom or wondering which of your kids will have to bunk together now that there's another cute human on the way. Regardless of your situation, know that God is the Father who provides. No one can outdo Him on that.

If you're wondering how you're going to make ends meet or get all of the gadgets you need, then understand that He cares for your unborn child even more than you do, and He wants nothing more than to provide them with everything they need. Stay in a position of gratitude knowing that God is working things out on your behalf.

List some things that God has provided for you and your baby that money can't buy. (For example, these things could include loving friends, a supportive partner, good health, etc.)

_____

_____

_____

_____

_____

_____

_____

What are some things that you've been worrying about that you can release to God today?

_____

_____

_____

_____

_____

_____

_____

_____

Write down some ways God has provided for you during this pregnancy that you didn't expect.

_____

_____

_____

_____

_____

_____

_____

Sometimes it feels like I don't have enough resources, help, or even space for my child on the way. Please make a way for those problems to be solved in Your strength, Father. (Continue your prayer here.)

_____

_____

_____

_____

_____

_____

_____

_____

Obstacles in the Way

> *"I have told you these things, so that in Me*
> *you may have peace. In this world*
> *you will have trouble. But take heart!*
> *I have overcome the world."*
>
> **JOHN 16:33 (NIV)**

Not everything goes according to plan in pregnancy or in life. Just ask Job, Moses, Noah, or pretty much anyone in the Bible. We are able to witness their trials through scripture, and they all dealt with their circumstances differently. The common thread among those in the Bible who never gave up despite their sufferings is that they relied on their faith in God. Jesus reminded us that we will face trouble in the world, but His promise was that He has already overcome the world.

No matter what situation you're facing, understand that God has already sent help and that's in Christ Himself. We can be encouraged that our Father already had foresight into what His children would face and didn't leave you to deal with it by yourself.

It might be tempting to avoid hardships or even pretend they won't happen, but accepting the difficulties that come with life is important because it also helps you acknowledge God in the midst of it. If we don't think we need His help, then we miss out on the blessing of having Him carry the burden for us.

Trust God to keep you and your child covered in His peace. Call out to Him for wisdom in any hard decisions you have to make during this time, and know that there is nothing you're going through that God can't handle. Keep reading stories of those who came out on the other side of their valleys with a testimony, and remember that He got them there. Keep your faith.

What types of struggles have you dealt with during this trimester, and how did God help you through them?

_____

_____

_____

_____

_____

_____

_____

Are there things you're facing that require you to really trust God? Be honest about your emotions dealing with this.

_____

_____

_____

_____

_____

_____

_____

_____

Write down a memory of something you've overcome in the past that can encourage you today.

_____

_____

_____

_____

_____

_____

_____

_____

_____

God, how can I release to You the intense emotions I have? (Continue your prayer here.)

_____

_____

_____

_____

_____

_____

_____

_____

_____

What's Your Motivation?

*Do nothing out of selfish ambition or vain conceit.
Rather, in humility value others above yourselves,
not looking to your own interests but each of you
to the interests of the others.*

PHILIPPIANS 2:3-4 (NIV)

My husband and I agreed when I was pregnant with my first child that we would hardly—if ever—post images of her on social media. This was to protect her privacy, because we didn't want tons of her images scattered online before she could give her permission.

However, once she was born, I couldn't help but post a photo of her adorable newborn face. The comments started rolling in, and I loved the feeling of having something *else* to do (like responding to those reactions), when nursing and recovering were practically the only things filling my days and nights.

Soon I was posting photos of her whenever I needed that emotional rush, completely forgetting about the agreement with my husband. Whoops. It actually took awhile (more than a year!) for me to understand that my desire to be seen outweighed anything else. My main focus was to get those interactions and for people to say how beautiful and unique my daughter was. Later on, I took down many of her pictures because of the selfish motivation behind my decision to post them.

God calls us to be humble and to do things not out of our own interests or vain conceit. There's nothing wrong with sharing your family or your cute pregnancy bump, but if your heart behind it is to get attention or to make yourself feel better, then please consider if it's doing more harm than good. Let us walk in humility and consider how our actions affect ourselves and others.

Have you felt like you needed to do things to get attention, just to make yourself feel better?

_____

_____

_____

_____

_____

_____

_____

Has being a mom made you feel more valuable or less valuable? Why or why not?

_____

_____

_____

_____

_____

_____

_____

_____

Describe a time after giving birth when you needed to feel validated by others.

_____

_____

_____

_____

_____

_____

_____

Lord, sometimes I'm crying out for attention from people. Please help me feel content from Your affection instead. (Continue your prayer here.)

_____

_____

_____

_____

_____

_____

_____

Emotion Explosion

We love because He first loved us.

1 JOHN 4:19 (NIV)

Some women take awhile to emotionally bond with their new-borns, whereas others fall in love immediately. Both scenarios are normal. With my daughter, I expected an instant connection, but it didn't happen. It actually took a few weeks for me to feel fully bonded. From the recovery of labor and delivery, to her scream-crying for the first few weeks of her life, and to the overall stress of adjusting to life as a mom, I just didn't have those ooh-aah feelings because I was so overwhelmed.

With my son it was much different. I felt in awe within the first few minutes and couldn't believe he was here and mine. Of course, I'm madly in love with both kids now. A mother's love for her children is almost indescribable. It's an explosion of feelings that prompts an instinctual "I would die for you."

Even though we feel that way, Jesus actually *did* it. He died for us because of His unconditional love. We know about love only because God showed us what it means in His word and through His son. Becoming a parent can bring so much more depth into our relationship with God.

In many ways motherhood strengthened my faith because I had to rely on Jesus like never before in my life. Parenting gave me the desperation to cling to Him because so much more is on the line. The next time you look into your child's eyes and feel like your heart might literally burst, remember that's how God feels about you.

Has your love for your baby deepened your understanding of just how much God loves you?

_____

_____

_____

_____

_____

_____

_____

_____

Were there any moments that made it harder to emotionally connect to your child?

_____

_____

_____

_____

_____

_____

_____

_____

_____

Write down the feelings you had right after giving birth. What were your initial thoughts about your child?

_____

_____

_____

_____

_____

_____

_____

_____

Thank you for sending Jesus to die for me and for reminding me of Your love through the love You've given me for my child. (Continue your prayer here.)

_____

_____

_____

_____

_____

_____

_____

_____

When Mama Bear Strikes

> *"Have I not commanded you? Be strong and courageous. Do not be afraid; do not be discouraged, for the Lord your God will be with you wherever you go."*
>
> **JOSHUA 1:9 (NIV)**

The first thing that you usually feel when bonding with your newborn is the intense heart-swelling love. Following that, many mothers discover a new boldness as the "mama bear" instincts rise up. Once my daughter was born, I remember being surprised by how quickly I defended myself and my baby whenever my parenting choices were criticized. I actually had to learn to tame what felt like a lion's roar being summoned at any moment.

This way of reacting may be new to you if you've been shy or not particularly outspoken in the past. If that's the case, then it's a great time to start praying about how to have balance in finding the courage God called us to have.

When you think of being courageous and strong, thoughtfully consider what that means for you personally. If you're used to always doing what other people tell you to do, then courage can be as simple as saying, "Okay, I'll think about it—thanks for your advice," instead of going along with it right away.

On the flip side, if you're often brash and your instinct is to immediately go into defense mode, then you can try a gentler approach to strength by learning to tame your tone, even if you disagree with someone.

Keep this in mind: You are one of the main advocates for you and your baby. Whatever the scenario, choose to do what will be best for your well-being and theirs, in a gentle and loving way.

List some ways you've found it hard to speak up on behalf of you or your child this past week.

_____

_____

_____

_____

_____

_____

_____

Are there any ways you can allow constructive criticism without becoming immediately defensive?

_____

_____

_____

_____

_____

_____

_____

_____

When was the first time you felt "mama bear" show up in your behavior since having your baby?

_____

_____

_____

_____

_____

_____

_____

Father, please help me stand up for myself and my family with boldness and also grace. (Continue your prayer here.)

_____

_____

_____

_____

_____

_____

_____

Keeping Up with Proverbs 31

*She watches over the affairs of her household and
does not eat the bread of idleness.*

PROVERBS 31:27 (NIV)

You may look at the woman in the well-known Proverbs 31 as the standard of what a mother does and how her day is run, but keep in mind that this passage outlines the characteristics of a woman after God's heart and not an exact template of what a Christian mom should do. Although you're probably getting up before the sun rises, it's most likely for another feeding and diaper change, not to make breakfast for your entire household.

Motherhood is a beautiful responsibility, but you can quickly feel like you're in way over your head. Becoming a multitasking mom takes time. You're not alone if some days are just too much, but there is definitely something to be said for developing a type of pattern and rhythm in your day; even if that pattern consists of feedings, making sure the Diaper Genie gets emptied before it starts to overflow, and changing your shirt that may or may not be covered in spit-up stains.

Ugh.

It's great to aspire to have everything under control one day.

But give yourself grace in the early days, knowing that sometimes keeping your household affairs in order is as simple as making sure everyone is safe and healthy. Check in with your support system to ensure your well-being is at the top of the to-do list as well.

List some ways you could use more help, and also jot down who in your support system you can ask to assist with those things.

_____

_____

_____

_____

_____

_____

_____

_____

Have you been actively making your well-being a priority? If so, then how? If not, then how can you change that?

_____

_____

_____

_____

_____

_____

_____

_____

As each day seems to bleed into the next, the newborn days can be a blur. Try to jot down one enjoyable memory that stood out to you this past week.

_____

_____

_____

_____

_____

_____

_____

Sometimes I want to be a "perfect mom." Lord, please help me extend grace to myself when I feel like I'm falling short. (Continue your prayer here.)

_____

_____

_____

_____

_____

_____

_____

_____

Just Wingin' It

> Trust in the Lord with all your heart and
> lean not on your own understanding; in all
> your ways submit to Him, and He will
> make your paths straight.
>
> **PROVERBS 3:5-6 (NIV)**

No matter how much research you've done, raising a child is mostly trial and error. Whether this is your first baby or your seventh, let's be honest: Most of us moms are out here just wingin' it. There's no playbook for being the perfect mother, but the best guidance we have to go on is the Word of God coupled with the Holy Spirit.

The motherhood journey should be an extension of your faith in God. It's not in a category of its own that can't be touched by God's presence. We know this because scripture reminds us to submit to God in *all* our ways. As much as social media would like you to believe that this one article or that one list of mommy tips and tricks is going to solve your problems, you'll be hard-pressed to find a better solution than going to God in prayer.

Of course, there are experts whose advice is helpful, but leaving God out of the equation can be detrimental to your self-esteem and confidence as a mom. Having faith in the latest "Mamas' Guide to Doing It All" can leave you feeling defeated when your baby doesn't respond to their guidance the way you thought they would.

The next time you're feeling tempted to keep up with every other mom, remember that your child is unique, so your approach to raising them will have to follow suit.

How much pressure have you put on yourself to live up to other people's expectations and results?

_____

_____

_____

_____

_____

_____

_____

What are some things you can do to alleviate the challenge of living up to someone else's standard?

_____

_____

_____

_____

_____

_____

_____

_____

Since having your baby, have you felt a difference between praying to God about how to handle motherhood challenges and seeking advice from someone else? Describe those differences.

_____

_____

_____

_____

_____

_____

Father, I know that You designed my child by hand. Please give me wisdom on the best way to take care of their needs. (Continue your prayer here.)

_____

_____

_____

_____

_____

_____

_____

_____

Sweet Like Honey

> *Gracious words are a honeycomb, sweet to the soul and healing to the bones.*
>
> **PROVERBS 16:24 (NIV)**

I had never heard of "mom shaming" until I joined a few online forums for mothers. Now that you're in bed with a newborn day and night, you have a lot of time to scroll, google, and scroll some more. Because of that, you've probably landed in one of these groups. Unfortunately, what should be a safe space to ask for advice often becomes a source of pain for many new and longtime moms.

During the months of your pregnancy, you inevitably thought a lot about the choices you'd make as a mom and the many reasons behind it. Sometimes, the lack of sleep and laundry piling up can turn even the softest mama into a harsh-toned mama bear—even if we don't intend it—when we project our own decisions onto other moms.

The truth is, every mother is just trying their best in the newborn days and beyond. This means we should offer more grace to others and even ourselves. When you find yourself judging someone or even talking down to yourself, remember the healing nature of a kind word.

Instead of telling another mom why you think her preference is wrong, take time to lift her up with all the things she's doing right. You might like things done a certain way around the house, but choose to thank your partner for their efforts in everything they do for you and your baby instead of critiquing them. Be quick to build up other people, as Jesus would do, and never forget to walk in love.

Has the advice or criticism from other people been hard for you to take during this newborn stage? Why or why not?

_____

_____

_____

_____

_____

_____

_____

Have you had a difficult time staying positive or saying uplifting things to other people right now? Why or why not?

_____

_____

_____

_____

_____

_____

_____

_____

List some times when you felt truly loved, understood, or supported this past week.

_____

_____

_____

_____

_____

_____

_____

_____

Father, I'm not always loving with my words, and sometimes I'm even judgmental of others. I need Your help in order to be better in lifting up others. (Continue your prayer here.)

_____

_____

_____

_____

_____

_____

_____

_____

The Good Stuff

> *Therefore, rid yourselves of all malice and all deceit, hypocrisy, envy, and slander of every kind. Like newborn babies, crave pure spiritual milk, so that by it you may grow up in your salvation, now that you have tasted that the Lord is good.*
>
> **1 PETER 2:1-3 (NIV)**

Newborns don't come out of the womb requesting a three-course dinner. Their sensitive tummies crave a simple breastmilk- or formula-only diet that can sustain them for months. So how is it that their brains can develop, their muscles can become strong, and their hair grows despite their meals being the same, day after day?

Newborns thrive because what we give them is the "good stuff," packed with every complex ingredient needed to sustain them. Even though breastmilk or formula looks simple to us, it contains every ingredient necessary for growth in all areas.

You might believe God can't offer you *everything* you need simply based on reading His word, talking to Him, and obeying His word. The Bible states that we should crave pure spiritual milk and do away with everything that doesn't serve us. Though you might be tempted to lean on a vice you've developed in venting to other people, complaining on social media, or comparing yourself with every other mom, don't keep that habit. It makes you feel good only on a temporary basis, but what God offers in a relationship with Himself sustains you in every area, leaving you feeling full and peaceful because it's designed just for you. He's got only the "good stuff."

Write down some moments when you've felt like God just "wasn't enough" for what you were going through.

_____

_____

_____

_____

_____

_____

_____

_____

Did finding solutions or happiness without Him ever yield the results you were looking for?

_____

_____

_____

_____

_____

_____

_____

_____

_____

Describe a time when you felt the closest to God during this "fourth trimester."

_____

_____

_____

_____

_____

_____

_____

_____

God, I know that You're enough, but sometimes it doesn't feel that way. Please help me get everything I need within my relationship with You. (Continue your prayer here.)

_____

_____

_____

_____

_____

_____

_____

_____

Acknowledgments

It's only by God's divine grace and inspiration that I've been able to find the words to encourage those who are embarking on such a special journey of faith in their pregnancy. The Holy Spirit gets credit for the words in this book because there is no way possible I could have written it in my own wisdom.

Furthermore, if it wasn't for my loving community that believes in my gift of sharing God's love through writing, then I might not have had the confidence to take on this important project.

I'd also like to thank my entire team at Rockridge Press of Callisto Media for entrusting me with the great responsibility of bringing this devotional to life. It couldn't have been made without your amazing support.

About the Author

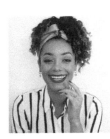

Kytia L'amour is a writer, performer, and public speaker spreading God's love in all art forms. The legacy she's leaving is teaching other people how they can find their identity in Christ and live a life of true freedom. She lives in sunny Southern California with her husband and children, where she's consistently creating thought-provoking content inspired by her relationship with Jesus Christ.